Evaluation of Clinical Reasoning Methods used by Junior Doctors in approaching patients with Leg Pain

By:

Dr Husam Ghazi Al-Anbari

(student number at University of Melbourne 748232)

Supervisors:

Dr Barbara Kameniar

Dr Jayne Lysk

Department of Medical Education
Melbourne Medical School - The University of Melbourne

November 2018

Abstract

Background:

It is agreed that diagnosis is at the heart of medicine. To make a diagnosis, health practitioners need a proper clinical reasoning approach and this is particularly complex in medical problems where chronic pain features. In general practice, junior practitioners face challenges such as time constraints, lack of experience, and dealing with a variety of medical problems. Pain is invisible and presents a challenging clinical reasoning and diagnostic problem. Although there is a large clinical reasoning education literature, less has been written about how to effectively teach clinical reasoning in general practice settings.

Objectives:

To explore *how* junior general practitioners clinically reason when treating patients with leg pain. To *critically analyse, my own* method of teaching clinical reasoning

Methods:

This study uses auto ethnographic methods. I wanted to describe and reflect on my own teaching of clinical reasoning. I was supervising **seven junior** General Practitioners in **two** different metropolitan general practices in Melbourne - Victoria in the period between 2015-2018. I had an opportunity to observe the students, record and describe what they did and how I taught them and then critically reflect on this process of learning and teaching. Based on this description and analysis, I introduced my own clinical reasoning method "Think Anatomy, Think Red Flags" and observed changes and recorded my reflections of the interactions and learning between the students and myself.

Results:

Most of junior general practitioners used an analytic hypothetical method of clinical reasoning. Yet, pain is a challenging medical problem and approaching this issue needs more experience and less reliance on structured hypothesis testing. Instead of directly teaching clinical reasoning, I came to understand I needed to focus on making my own expertise and experience visible to the students. I focused on encouraging students to "Think Anatomy; Think Red Flags" as this represented my own way of thinking.

Discussion and Conclusions:

Although the analytic hypothetic method of clinical reasoning is the most widely used method for learning and teaching clinical reasoning, this auto ethnographic study highlighted the need to orient students towards particular features and mechanisms of pain to more effectively assist them to develop reasoning skills. The research showed the importance of *individualising* clinical reasoning methods to each medical specialties. Based on close observations of both student learning and my own teaching, I developed the "Think Anatomy Think Red Flags" model

Keywords:
Clinical Reasoning, Pain, General Practice, Think Anatomy Think Red Flags

Acknowledgements

First and foremost, I would like to express my sincere gratitude to my supervisors Dr Barbara Kameniar and Dr Jayne Lysk, for their professional advice and guidance, patience, enthusiasm, motivation and intense knowledge. I would like to thank A/Prof. Clare Denaly for encouraging my research and for your brilliant comments and suggestions.

Finally, I would like to thank my family and friends, especially my parents and my wife (Nuha), words cannot express how grateful I am. Thank you for unwavering support of my decision to pursue graduate education and for all the sacrifices you have made on my behalf. Your prayer for me was what sustained me thus far. To my daughters Amenah and Zahraa and my son Mohammed, and *the coming fourth son (Mehdi)!* for enduring life with a graduate student father, I love you dearly. My friends that I have been blessed with since my arrival to Melbourne, thank you for your caring and support.

Contents

1.0 Introduction
1.1 What is Clinical Reasoning?

1.2 What is General Practice?

1.3 Literature Review of Clinical Reasoning Methods used in General Practice

2.0 Methodology

2.1 Introduction

2.2 Auto ethnography Methodology

2.3 Action Research Methodology

2.4 My Journey of Teaching Clinical Reasoning

3.0 Results - Contextualising The problem

3.1 Introduction

3.2 Some of my Observations

3.3 Trainees' Clinical Approaches

3.4 Think Anatomy Think Red Flags- Heuristic Approach

3.5 My Model and Other Models

3.6 Few Examples After Teaching "Think Anatomy Think Red Flags" Model

4.0 Discussion

4.1 Discussing Clinical Reasoning Methods

4.2 Discussing My Results in Comparison to Others

5.0 Conclusion

6.0 References

1.0 INTRODUCTION

1.1 What is Clinical Reasoning?

Many different terms have been used to describe clinical reasoning such as problem solving or clinical judgment, clinical diagnosis or diagnostic reasoning and clinical decision-making. However, clinical reasoning is the term most used to describe the thinking processes used by medical and health professionals to understand clinical problem/s and try to treat it/them accordingly (Higgs 2008, Findyartini 2012, Vallente 2016). Some authors have stated that clinical reasoning is an essential skill for future teaching and learning (Ilgen et al. 2012). Clinical reasoning might be understood as a form of critical thinking (Atkinson et al. 2011; Delany and Golding 2014; Vallente 2016). Students usually find clinical reasoning difficult because it is a complex and difficult skill to define and, as a form of thinking internal to an expert, it is invisible to students (Delany & Golding 2014). As a result, it has been argued that clinicians working with students should assist them by making their thinking processes visible. Delany and Golding suggested a number of strategies for use by clinical educators to assist them in helping students to understand and practice clinical reasoning (Delany and Golding 2014). Some of these tools are:

Advise students to make a plan for collecting data.

Find out the justifications for the clinical judgment.

Simplify the tasks.

Give feedback to students.

Teach students how to match ideas and reach conclusions.

Encourage them to use common sense in clinical reasoning.

What can a clinical teacher do to help students to develop their clinical reasoning skills?

Clinical educators usually try to assist students to identify their ways of thinking and this is achieved through a number of different approaches including:

- The delivery of more teaching (lectures, case based discussions and other forms of clinical educations). This allows students to have more exposure to a variety of clinical challenges which enhance experience (Delany and Golding 2014).
- The provision of feedback. Students need to know more about the quality of their performance including mistakes or good performance Feedback is vital in reshaping students' ways of thinking and it enhances the possibility they will achieve a better approach in critical thinking (Molloy and Boud 2014).
- Opportunities for observation Students can watch their teachers while they approach patients and learn from this opportunity. This enables teachers to demonstrate their approach and show students some of the requisite skills. In this way, students will have the opportunity to improve skills and approach patients (Higgs 2008, Delany and Golding 2014)
- Thinking out loud. Clinical teachers can express their thinking "out

loud" by openly articulating their thinking strategies or techniques so students can learn clearly and effectively and teachers will make their thinking "visible" (Delany and Molloy 2009).

- Peer Observations. Encourage students to watch each others and then critique each other. The teacher's role in this approach is to be the coordinator because this will help each one understand and explore others' skills and with time will lead to more knowledge and skills (Macrum 2018).

Clinical reasoning is considered routine to anyone working in health practice, and experienced practitioners use it automatically (Elstein et al. 1981, Findyartini 2012, Levine and Bleakley 2013). Elstein et al. (1981) propose that clinical reasoning has a number of steps which need to be followed to optimise the health service. These steps include: collect information from the patient, analyse the information, recognise the challenges, set aims, plan management, review outcomes and finally incorporate the results of the management into future learning teaching processes.

Clinical reasoning is not a simple process since health practitioners encounter different medical challenges that make using clinical reasoning in solving one issue not enough to solve the next because each patient and context is different. Hence medical practitioners need a considerable amount of knowledge to use clinical reasoning effectively (McBee et al. 2015).

1.2 What is general Practice?

The Royal Australian College of General Practitioners (RACGP) described general practice as a method of delivering the patients, their relatives and the community with a safe comprehensive, patient centered health care (Gardner and Mazza 2012; Khalil and Schliephake 2017).

The RACGP set certain clinical curriculum which reflects the guidelines of proper health practice within five domains:

Domain 1 - Communication skills and the patient-doctor relationship (e.g. communication skills, patient centred, health promotion, whole person care)

Domain 2 – Applied professional knowledge and skills (e.g. physical examination and procedural skills, medical conditions, decision making).

Domain 3 – Population health and the context of general practice (e.g. epidemiology, public health, prevention, family influence on health, resources).

Domain 4 – Professional and ethical role (e.g. duty of care, standards, self appraisal, teacher role, research, self care, networks)

Domain 5 – Organisational and legal dimensions (e.g. information technology, records, reporting, confidentiality, practice management) (Gardner and Mazza 2012, Morgan, Ingham et al. 2015, Khalil and Schliephake 2017).

This study will be a reflection of my teaching in two metropolitan general practices. In these practices there are seven general practitioners under training.

From the above five domains, I will focus on the second one which is how to cultivate professional knowledge and skills by using appropriate clinical reasoning to enhance correct decision making.

In general practice, the diagnosis of any medical problems is considered the most essential step (Linn et al. 2012). General practitioners, unlike some other specialties such as surgeons, consult with patients on a daily basis and they follow sequential steps in diagnosis, namely taking a patient's history then performing a physical examination and finally requesting investigations accordingly before reaching a diagnosis and proposing treatment (Norman et al. 2014, Shahram et al. 2017). Diagnosis is at the heart of medical work and to reach it, the health practitioner must use clinical reasoning. For this reason, it is agreed that teaching clinical reasoning is a fundamental stage in clinical education (Levine and Bleakley 2013).

General practitioners face many more challenges in diagnosing medical problems in comparison to other specialties because they must explore all aspects of the patient at an early stage of presentation while other specialists such as neurologists will focus on more specific aspects. Additionally, general practitioners deal with more uncertainty than others (Chew-Graham and May 1999, Downs et al. 2004). General practitioners also usually consult quite a large number of patients in a shorter time frame than other specialists (Chew-Graham and May 1999).

Over the last few decades, there has been a considerable focus in the literature on studying clinical reasoning. This has added more to our knowledge, however, the main focus has tended to be on comparing a beginners' and an experts' capacity to use clinical reasoning (Norman 2005, Monteiro and Norman 2013). There has been a lack of studying clinical reasoning in the field of general practice and a number of other specialties (Yazdani et al. 2017).

1.3 Literature Review of Clinical Reasoning Methods in General Practice

This section of the study explores a range of literature before critically reviewing different models of clinical reasoning. The focus will be on the use of clinical reasoning in general practice. As stated above, clinical reasoning can be expressed with many synonyms such as diagnostic reasoning, problem solving skills, clinical judgment or diagnostic strategies. In this study the term clinical reasoning will be used to simplify the task. A brief discussion on each of the models follows:

1. Hypothetical – deductive clinical reasoning (analytic)

This approach of clinical reasoning depends largely on an analytic way of medical problem solving. Clinicians facing a medical problem commence by consulting the patient and collecting all necessary information before producing a number of hypotheses (ideas). With time they might produce more questions / hypotheses in response to new data collection and so on then the clinicians will include or exclude (deduct) some of these ideas before coming to a final decision or diagnosis of the problem. This method has been described by Elstein and colleagues (1981) (Elstein 2009, Atkinson et al. 2011).

The major features of this method are:
- Collection of information from systematic history taking, performing physical examinations and gathering other evidence from patient documents.
- Mental processing of the information. This step varies from one to another depending on mental capacity and level of experience in the field of medicine.
- Clinicians creating a plan of management according to the available data.

2. Pattern Recognition Method (Non Analytic) of clinical reasoning

This method was described by Arocha and colleagues (1993) who argued that there is a method of clinical diagnosis which involves clinicians recognising a diagnosis by utilizing pattern recognition (Arocha et al. 1993). This process of thinking happens when the clinicians encounter the patients, they use all possible clues (from history taking or physical examinations or available records) and arrange them in a pattern to reach the diagnosis (Norman et al. 2007). This method is largely dependent on previous knowledge and skills. It is quicker than the hypothetic deductive method since the clinicians will not proceed with all steps of that clinical approach. When the clinicians encounter new medical presentations, they use their memory and compare the new ones with the "model" or "prototype" or old presentations and match the new with the most appropriate prototype presentation to reach a diagnosis and final management plan (Monteiro and Norman 2013).

3. Dual Clinical Reasoning

This clinical reasoning model has been described by Croskerry (2009) who integrated the two above methods of clinical reasoning (analytic and non analytic methods) into a single approach (Croskerry, 2009). In this approach, the clinicians use both methods to reach a clinical diagnosis and treatment. They use non analytic ways of thinking, when appropriate to reach a diagnosis and finalise their management. Otherwise, the analytic method (Eva 2002) will be the second option to be applied. This method of reasoning is much more flexible than others since it gives more freedom to the clinician to use the best available method of thinking. The analytic method helps to minimize some of the potential mistakes of non analytic – pattern recognition approaches (Higgs

2008, Findyartini 2012, Linn et al. 2012).

4. **Pathway for Clinical Reasoning**

During the patients' consultations, clinicians have a group of questions that include establishing the patient's current presentation as well as probing into the patient's past health and family history. From the answers to those questions, clinicians navigate their way to a more specific exploration of the needed questions and cues. The clinicians gather the most relevant data and ignore the more detailed questions or data which are considered as time consuming or irrelevant. This method of clinical reasoning was examined by Ribeiro and colleagues (2010) who found that if clinicians fail to reach a conclusion from the available information, they usually explore more evidence and examine more hypotheses. This method is a trial of utilising the available data as much as possible but without following the routine analytic methods of clinical reasoning.

5. **Clinical (Diagnostic) Reasoning Strategies Method**

The clinical reasoning strategies method was described by Balla et al (2009). The cardinal feature of this model is the use of three stages. In each stage there are a number of strategies (Balla, Heneghan et al. 2009).

The three stages:

Firstly, generate a diagnostic hypothesis. This stage has a few strategies such as:

- spot diagnosis for instance a patient with skin rash of Herpes Zoster pattern. In this scenario, the clinician will be able to diagnose the patient by inspecting the lesion, however s/he will ask more questions to clarify the underlying causes or other related clinical problems

- Self diagnosis, when patients tell clinicians about their story which gives reasons and diagnosis, for instance a female patient with recurrent urinary tract infection can express her symptoms and mostly she knows her problem which will help a clinician to establish an hypothesis.

Secondly, refine this hypothesis, during which a few strategies can be used such as:

- Forward clarification of the problem by asking more questions or ordering more investigations.

- Probabilistic reasoning is one of the strategies (Kostopoulou et al. 2008; Findyartini 2012) that can be used efficiently in this mode. For example, the age of the patient can predict the diagnosis. If the clinicians face a patient under 10 years of age with back pain, they will not think of degenerative disease since osteoarthritis is unlikely to happen during this age, but may consider child abuse or an injury from a fall. In this scenario, the probability will play an essential role in diagnosis. Despite this strategy being helpful with some diagnoses, it might fail to help in some other medical conditions when the probability cannot be of help, for instance, a 40-year-old man with a non-specific headache. In this scenario there will be wide range of possibilities and a physician should use many steps and strategies to identify the problem.

Thirdly, outline the final diagnosis. This can be achieved by analysing all available data and integrating them with the clinicians' past experience and skills to reach the final diagnosis.

This method of clinical reasoning is designed to utilise both analytic and non-analytic clinical reasoning methods but the differentiating characteristic of this method is using the strategies which enable clinicians to move freely from analytic to non-analytic methods in a flexible manner (Emanovský 2015).

6. An Integrative method of clinical reasoning

In the integrative method of clinical reasoning model, the authors examined some features to enable the clinician to solve the clinical problem. They suggested that there are at least two cardinal sources of information which can lead to initial representation. These features are the medical practitioners' past information about the patients and the patients' clinical presentations. The clinicians will examine these two sources and might reach the diagnosis but if they cannot, they will reassess the findings and try to collect more evidence. They can repeat this process many times until finding the solution of the medical problem so they follow cycles of clinical work (Norman et al. 2002).

2.0 METHODOLOGY

2.1 Introduction

This study was conducted in two main metropolitan general practice clinics in Victoria - Australia. My role is supervisor to trainee doctors who are junior and in the first or second year of their training. I used qualitative methods in this study which are auto ethnography and action research. I observed my trainees' clinical reasoning approach and recorded my data then introduced a new model of clinical reasoning and recorded any changes in my trainees' clinical approach.

This chapter will be structured into three main sections:

- Auto ethnography Methodology
- Action Research Methodology
- My Story of Teaching Clinical Reasoning

2.1 Auto ethnography Methodology

Auto ethnography is a qualitative research method used in many knowledge fields such as Physiotherapy, the Arts, Education, Anthropology, Social Work, Psychology and within any field where the self-reflections of the researcher are considered a valuable and revealing part of the research process (Ellis et al. 2010, Adams et al. 2015, Borders and Giordano 2016, Chang 2016).

Auto ethnography is best understood by examining the meaning of the various root components of the word "Auto- Ethno-Graphy". Auto means self, Ethno means culture and Graphy means writing. In auto ethnography, the writer utilises self-reflection to record self-observations. They then link these to broader educational, social or cultural implications (Ellis et al. 2011, Adams et al. 2015).

When we try to explore a few details about the history of auto ethnography, we find that around the late 20th century and after the initial influence of postmodern ideas, there were more inquiries by social scientists to answer (Ellis et al. 2010). This enabled them to deliver much important information about the processes of the research and the researcher's role in interpreting what they encountered, rather than only write theories. Auto ethnography started to be used widely among researchers in many fields of knowledge such as social scientists, politicians, communication, education and more (Ellis et al. 2010, Adams et al. 2015, Egeli 2017).

Auto ethnography might be defined as a qualitative research method which enables a researcher to explore certain groups of people or culture or phenomenon and record self observations (Ellis et al. 2010, Hogan 2013, Adams et al. 2015, Chang 2016). Ellis (2010) defined auto ethnography as a method by which the researchers can describe and write (graphy) their own reflection (auto) so as to comprehend cultural awareness (ethno) (Ellis et al. 2010).

Many scholars found that people have a wide diversity in belief, experience, emotion and many other aspects of humanity. This led to concluding the real need of exploring this diversity and to record observations and analyse them (Ellis et al. 2010, Hogan 2013, Racine 2016, Egeli 2017).

Forms of Auto ethnography

The achievement of auto ethnographic work depends on many factors:
- The level of the writer's attention to people's stories.
- The quality of the self reflection or interactions with the community or interviewing others.
- Depth of analysis of data.
- How to engage methods of research and the writer's scientific background?
- How to apply all of these within the community (Ellis, Adams et al. 2011).

There are many forms of auto ethnography including Indigenous, narrative and reflexive approaches (Ellis et al. 2010, Hogan 2013, Adams et al. 2015).

- Indigenous, when some people uses ethnography to explain their own personal or cultural experience with no much analysis.
- Narrative, when ethnographers tell stories of others with no detailed analysis.
- Reflexive when ethnographers record data, analyse them and present them after engaging their own scientific background as researchers (Ellis et al 2010).

Some proponents have suggested ethnography can be part of a solution to certain community issues. This can be well applied if the author succeeds in engaging his/her personal observation/ story with the community's problem or need and might end up with opening a window to a solution (Racine 2016, Egeli 2017).

In my thesis I will describe how I observed the reactions of trainee general practitioners to the specific problem of "a patient with leg pain" and then will reflect on that and present my records aiming to improve general practitioners' clinical reasoning skills and performance or at least providing a foundation for future study. Hence, I am using reflexive type of auto ethnography.

Privacy and Auto ethnography

When telling a story, we often need to mention the story's participants and circumstances, places, time and other events to make the story engaging and realistic. However, this might lead to disclosing others' opinions, views, belief and other personal issues. This might interfere with the privacy of others which can threaten researchers' work and affects their professional relationships for instance when an author writes some details about a group of people this might lead to disclosure of this group's identity which will breach their privacy. For that reason and to avoid this problem, it is recommended for any ethnographer to avoid frank statements about any discussions or situations which might have direct clues to some people (Ellis et al. 2010).

In my thesis, I will use a few strategies such as:
- Trainees will be labeled as trainee 1 (T1), trainee 2 (T2) and so on to minimise them being identified.
- Patients will be mentioned without names or date of birth or any specific clues which might help identify them.
- Details about each patient will be brief to avoid breaching privacy.
- No direct quotation of statements of patients or trainees will be used as this thesis is primarily concerned with my reflections.

Auto ethnography and Critiques

There are a number of criticisms about auto ethnography as a method of research. Some of these include:
- Auto ethnography depends largely on self expression which is considered by Sparkes (2000) as an issue of conflict, since auto ethnographers emphasise self reflection and this lack of objectivity might produce bias (Sparkes 2000).
- Other critics consider auto ethnographers to be narcissistic, showing excessive interest in themselves. While other critics have argued that auto ethnographers do not put in the requisite effort to justify important conclusions that might be found when using large data.

> For example, auto ethnographers collect data from observations only, record and interpret their observations and this is not sufficient as a scientific method of research (Atkinson 1997; Méndez 2013).
- Walford (2004) expressed concern about how auto ethnographers write up their research through the telling of their stories. He argues that writing a story is not research (Walford 2004; Méndez 2013).
- Additionally, some critics argue that auto ethnographers are self-reflecting only and they might be biased because of that, since they will include their own ideas and beliefs into their story (Hogan 2013).

On the other side, Ellis and colleagues (2011) argue that using self narratives is a helpful tool as they give an auto ethnographer the opportunity to reflect on his or her personal experience in recording and analysing collected data (Ellis, Adams et al. 2011).

In Auto ethnography, the writers will not only describe things but analyse them (Ellis et al. 2010, Adams et al. 2015, Borders and Giordano 2016). It is essential that the author plays a role of community participant observer to watch closely and describe observations clearly and by doing that, the auto ethnographer is aiming to help the community members to better understand their culture/community and at the same time, those who are outside that community can look and understand that community better (Ellis et al. 2010, Hogan 2013, Chang 2016). The most interesting thing about auto ethnographers is that they are not merely story tellers but rather, they are researchers and have their own methods, theories and scientific background which enables them to watch, record and analyse their recording and present that as their results of study in a trustworthy way (Ellis et al. 2010).

Auto ethnographers must be able to describe things in a sophisticated and in-depth way while telling their story because this will engage readers or learners to interact positively with the content of what they are saying and support the trustworthiness of their account. Additionally, the writer should be capable of engaging the readers with the story applying multiple methods such as writing an interview or a consultation or real stories which might be readily understandable to readers and enable them to live the situation (Ellis et al. 2010; Adams et al. 2015).

The writer might use "I" as first person to illustrate some observations, however it might be accepted to use second or third person to describe certain events. It is all about how well an auto ethnographer presents his/her work to readers or learners (Ellis et al. 2010).

In my thesis, I had enough time to record my observations, interact directly with my students and analyse my data and then engage my scientific background and educational theories to end up with results and conclusions. I critically discussed my results and concluded with some recommendations in a scientific way.

Someone helped me!

I was inspired to use auto ethnography by Prof Ali Al-Wardi (1913-1995) one of Iraq's social scientists who studied in the USA and came back to Iraq in 1950 to establish a new approach to understanding Iraqi culture. My maternal grandmother was talking to me about him when I was a child because he is her cousin, and she was telling me he studied abroad and established a solid education system in Baghdad University and there is a hall in this University named after him as a remembrance. Prof Al-Wardi described his approach to research in one of his TV interviews. He said, "I sit with lay people in a cafe or any place and talk to them in their simple language then I record their ideas and analyse that and present in writing to readers". He added, "I do not read people from books rather I write books from people's stories".

I was inspired by his approach and what he presented to Iraqi culture, and when I was doing this thesis I noticed that for the first time I am using his approach to analyse my data and present them in academic educational work. I believe it is rewarding to understand ourselves and our students using an auto ethnographic approach.

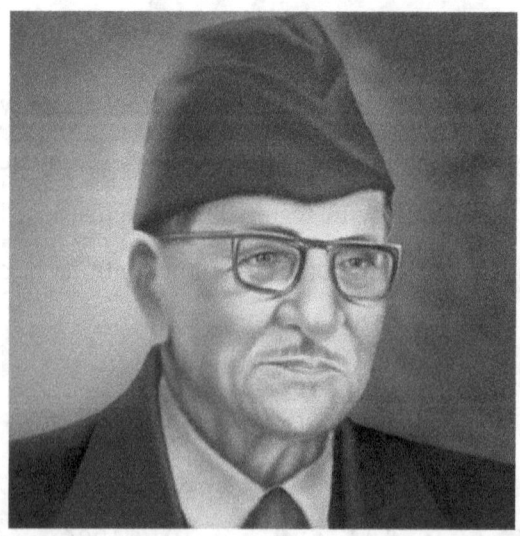

Figure (1) Prof. Ali Al-Wardi - Iraqi Social Scientist
Prof. Ali Al-Wardi (https://en.wikipedia.org/wiki/Ali_Al-Wardi)

2.2 Action Research Methodology

To provide a structure for the auto ethnography, I utilised an action research methodology.

What is Action Research?

Action research is a meticulous qualitative method of examination guided by and for those performing the study. The main aim of action research is to improve the environment of the practice. It is a type of self-reflection in which everyone can reflect and then develop the workplace. Action research is widely used in educational organisations but it is not commonly used in clinical practice, unless in clinical education. Some authors consider action research is just like an experiment when the researcher performs some tests and watches the result then responds accordingly. In education study, the researcher can implement some actions with learners then examine the response and reflect on that before undertaking a new action (Efron 2013, McAteer 2013).

What is the purpose of action research?

Action research in this thesis focuses on three main purposes:
- Building a thoughtful doctor.
- Making progress in clinical education culture.
- Improving the professional environment (McAteer 2013).

How can I do action research study?

Usually there are a few steps to follow while thinking about implementing this type of research in any study. The following steps are recommended:
1. Try to find the subject that will be examined. In any educational challenge, there are many areas of interest, the teacher or researcher needs to find the most influential aspects to explore and plan for this exploration (Efron 2013). In this study, the subject under examination is the use of clinical reasoning in general practice.
2. Identifying the underlying concepts of the specific subject that the researcher wants to examine. In this study, I reviewed literature dealing with clinical reasoning and its implication in clinical work especially for general practitioners (Efron 2013, McAteer 2013, McNiff 2017).
3. The next step is to clarify the research question as the researcher decides the subject and reviews others' work (McNiff 2017).

The questions in this instance are:
- To *explore how* junior general practitioners clinically reason when treating patients with leg pain.
- To *critically analyse, methods of teaching clinical reasoning*

4. Gathering Records by collecting data from the study, however it is essential to ensure that they are trustworthy (Efron 2013, McNiff 2017). The gathering in this thesis will only be the self reflections of the researcher in relationship to their interactions with trainees. I will use both auto ethnography and action research so I will utilise the area of intersection of both methods.
5. Examining the records. That is, after collecting them, it is the time to analyse them. In action research, there is no need for more sophisticated

statistical methods of analysis. Analysis depends on answering this question: 'What is the story of these observations and findings and what can be learned from these observations and findings?' If the researcher can find the story and tell it to others, it will be the best method in action research (Efron 2013, Stringer 2014). In this study I looked at my observations and analysed them.

6. Reporting Outcomes. It is challenging to define the results in this study as the researcher is both the researcher and the reporter and the results will solely depend on his or her interpretations (Stringer 2014; McNiff 2017). In my study, I was able to record my results and present them as outcomes and conclusions of my work.

7. Delivering an action. It is recommended for any action research project that findings should not only be presented but also actioned. It is the heart of any action research project to help others understand more about the subject of the study and look forward for further development (Efron 2013, Stringer 2014). After close observations of my students' performance, I was able to deliver an action which was teaching them another clinical approach to patients with leg pain and that was new model.

2.3 My Journey of Teaching Clinical Reasoning

This section of the chapter commences my narrative. I will give my auto ethnographic observations as a story about doing my teaching in a clinical setting. As noted above, I used action research to provide a structure to my teaching and observations of responses of the trainees to that teaching.

There is an interesting story that I lived while approaching many challenges in teaching clinical reasoning. I have to confess that it is my first time to use this auto ethnographic method in writing a thesis however I found it useful and promising.

Where and whom to teach!

The study is based in two metropolitan general practice clinics in Victoria where I teach seven general practitioners who are under training during a period between 2015-2018. However, I also teach in other places as I am currently undertaking training in pain management and interventions. I had an opportunity to meet general practitioners in their work place as well as in some lecture areas where I give some teaching to them as part of my role in training.

What to teach and why?

I know that general practitioners are dealing with nearly every medical aspect of their patients so they face a wide range of challenges. In particular, understanding and approaching a patient with pain is sometimes very difficult depending on the context of presentation of patients. One of the common presentations of the patients in general practice is leg pain.

I chose this subject "clinical approach to patients with leg pain" because:
- It is common.
- I have spent quite a lot of time in pain management so I have extensive experience in managing this medical challenge.
- I have found from my own experience that it can be challenging sometimes.
- The pain might arise from different causes (Murtagh and

Rosenblatt 2015).
- The pain tends to be chronic.
- Pain is invisible (it is subjective not objective) which adds more stress on doctors to come up with a diagnosis and management plan, and on the patient to be able to describe the pain in such a way that it assists the doctor.
- I have to limit my scope of observation so I can focus on one of the examples of clinical reasoning and learn more by observation.

Leg Pain

Pain in legs might include any pain from the hips to the toes. It might be the result of something simple such as a sprain or something serious such as cancer of the bone. Diagnosis of leg pain can be as easy as only inspecting the area and finding the reason such as in herpes zoster pain when the doctor can see herpes vesicles. However, it might need much more sophisticated investigations such as lumbo-sacral MRI (Magnetic resonance imaging) to diagnose nerve root compression in the lumbar spine region.

There are many reasons for leg pain and many different classifications of pain in the legs. Some health practitioners prefer pathological classification where they depend on types of diseases such as (infections, vascular, neoplastic, metabolic …etc), others might prefer anatomical classifications such as (nerve, bone, ligament, muscle …etc), and some prefer to classify it as radicular pain (coming from low back origin) or non radicular (when it arises from the legs).

Each one has his/her own clinical approach in classifying medical problems that can lead to leg pain. However, the clinical reasoning required to diagnose the causes of leg pain depends on almost the same principles as outlined in the review of literatures when medical practitioners use one or more of the clinical reasoning approaches described above (Yazdani et al. 2017).

Generally speaking, clinical reasoning depends on many factors including personal experience, the context of the clinical challenge, the setting or place (hospital vs private consulting room), age of patients and many other factors (Murtagh and Rosenblatt 2015).

Let me give an example: a 45-year-old gentleman presented with leg pain after lifting a heavy object a few days ago. The pain was sharp and moved from his back to right leg and up to his foot. In this scenario, the medical practitioner will usually focus in his clinical approach on radicular nerve pain which means the origin of pain is from the back and it moved to the right leg. The practitioner will need further study to prove or disprove his/her provisional diagnosis and will order tests such as Magnetic Resonance Imaging (MRI). This is mostly an analytic clinical reasoning model which is commonly used by health practitioners (Yazdani et al. 2017).

Another example is a 17-year-old female high school student who presented with ankle pain after participating in some sport activities at school. I think the first impression of any medical practitioner when approaching this patient would be that the ankle is sprained, however, it might be something else such as a fracture or infection. In this instance, s/he should take careful history including any past medical history and undertake proper clinical examination.

The case might need some investigations.

Now, what is next?

After observing the trainees doing their job while approaching patients with leg pain and there were mainly using analytic method of clinical reasoning, I introduced a new clinical reasoning approach. This new clinical approach is called: *Think Anatomy, Think Red Flags*.

I developed this clinical reasoning method after many years of working in the management of chronic pain and by observing many medical practitioners including my students. It is derived from an anatomical approach used in the classification of diseases and involves paying unique attention to the most serious or rare conditions.

Think Anatomy comes first because most health practitioners start their approach to patients with taking history and while they do that they start thinking (*what* is the problem?). So this approach will fit their thinking in a more organised fashion when they ask themselves "*where* is the problem: does the pain come from bone, muscle, joint, ligament, tendon, nerve, vessels (artery or vein), subcutaneous tissue or skin?". These are the anatomical structures in leg.

Then move to the **second part which is: Think Red Flags**, because anyone might miss serious or rare medical conditions such as cancer, thyroid disorder, depression, the side effects of medications or recreational drugs, Multiple sclerosis, paraneoplastic disease (cancer is somewhere else while patients complain a neurological deficit in another part of the body), mental issues (depression or others), chronic regional pain syndrome CRPS or something else.

3.0 RESULTS - Contextualising The Problem

3.1 Introduction

In this chapter I will outline some basic methods of teaching in a clinical setting before setting out the findings.

A clinical teacher might deliver teaching in a range of modes, these might include:

- The teacher is an observer while a student presents his/her performance, for instance, a student can take a history from a patient and, in the first instance, the teacher merely observes. Afterwards the teacher will interview the student, provide feedback, and have a discussion with them.
- A student performing an examination on a simulated patient or performing a simulated skilled procedure while the teacher supervises directly and intervenes when necessary (Adamson and Kardong-Edgren 2012).
- A student presents his or her performance to a teacher without the patient being present. This can be done in a group teaching situation where the teacher can engage other students in discussion (Collins and Harden 1998, Issenberg et al. 2011).

These are some of the main situations of teaching in a clinical work place. However, there might be other methods such as phone calls, discussions, emails or lecture presentations.

It is essential to mention that all trainee doctors mentioned in this study were junior and in the first or second year of their training.

3.2 Some of My Observations

The following will be samples from my records/data which can be used as a good reflection of my observations. I tried to avoid repetitions of similar findings for that reason I mentioned only samples of data.

Story number 1: (My left leg is annoying me, it is hot!)   How to approach?

An 81-year-old gentleman presented with a history of left leg discomfort of few months ago.
One of the general practitioners (Trainee 1= T1) consulted this patient and I was in another room. Afterwards we had a discussion and the patient came later and we (T1 and I) consulted him together.

Patient's clinical history:
The patient presented with left leg discomfort and the sensation of the leg being hot. He noted, "My left leg is annoying, it is hot". According to the patient the leg was (hot?) like few months ago but this happened progressively. He has hypertension, hyperlipidemia, and chronic neck and lower back pain. He had cervical spine surgery 10 years ago.
T1 took a clinical history and did a physical examination for this patient. T1 finished the consultation and the patient left. T1 came into my room and we

had a discussion.

T1 presented the history and clinical examination findings in a systematic way starting from the patient's details (name, age and gender) then main complaint with a history of the present illness then past medical history, mental and social history, then clinical examination findings and finally, results from any relevant medical investigations. Then T1 came up with a plan of management.

My observations

I noticed T1 was very keen to mention many details from the conversation with the patient. Some of those details were irrelevant, possibly because T1 does not like to miss anything or this is the method of clinical presentation T1 had learned in medical schools.

T1 was affected by the patient's first statement "my leg is hot" and I noticed T1 was focusing on the clinical features and causes of a leg that is hot. That is, T1 was focused on the *what* of the presentation.

It was very impressive how T1 was organised in mentioning the differential diagnoses of this presentation. T1 thought it might be peripheral neuropathy. However, T1 missed the opportunity to examine and compare the temperature of both legs because the left leg was not hot, it was actually of normal temperature but the right leg was cold because it was an ischaemic leg, and T1 missed examining peripheral pulses. That is, T1 omitted to focus on the *where* of the heat or pain origin.

This patient had a right ischemic limb because when I saw him (later) I noticed the right leg was cold in comparison to the left. This was confirmed by the use of a non-touch thermometer and by feeling the peripheral pulse. I found both legs had diminished pulses but mostly the right leg. I ordered an arterial

Doppler which showed almost complete occlusion of the right femoral artery with incomplete occlusion of the left femoral artery. I referred him to a vascular surgeon.

What did we learn?

A hot leg comes mostly with neuropathic pain. For that reason, I think T1 was driven to peripheral neuropathy. When I finished the discussion with T1, I recognised T1 agreed that there was a missing part in her clinical approach which is at least to compare and to remember vascular insult as part of differential diagnoses and not to adhere solely to a patient's words since in this scenario the patient's description was misleading.

This story represents a type of trainee doctor who uses Hypothetical – deductive clinical reasoning (analytic) as a default clinical approach. The clinicians will face the medical problem by consulting the patients then they produce a few hypotheses (ideas) after collecting all necessary information. With time they might produce more questions / hypotheses in response to new data collection and so on then the clinicians will include or exclude (deduct) some of these ideas to come to a final decision. This method is mainly described by Elstein et al (1981) (Elstein 2009, Shulman et al. 1981, Atkinson et al. 2011).

Story Number 2: "My Right half numb with needles sensation"

A 37-year-old man presented with a history of right side body numbness and the sensation of pins-and-needles in both his right arm and leg but with no numbness in face. The symptoms were localised to the area around the elbow and knee joints to a stage that he could not feel any sensation in these particular areas. There was no other complaint. This condition started suddenly but progressed to the stage that he was scared he had a stroke.

The patient was known to have chronic lower back pain. He has a history of pilonidal sinus surgery, is not diabetic or hypertensive. He also has a history of anxiety/Post traumatic stress disorder.

This patient was seen by trainee 2 (T2). This patient is known to me. He has visited me for about 4 years for chronic pain.

T2 took a clinical history and performed a clinical examination before discussing a plan of management.

T2 faced many difficulties such as: the patient was jumping in history taking from one subject to another and accusing previous doctors of mistreating him. He thought all of his problems were because of the delay in pilonidal surgery and he wanted to recover to where he was seven years ago.

T2 discovered this patient had a neurological complaint which cannot be explained with any anatomical pattern and cannot be understood well.

My observations

I discussed this condition with T2 who described this case as one of the *most difficult cases in whole training*. T2 was quite successful in obtaining a detailed history from the patient. While performing clinical examinations, T2 could not identify any anatomical relationship of patient's complaint and for that reason T2 came to the conclusion that it was a psychosomatic problem and preferred to send him to a psychologist.

I noticed when a clinical presentation of any patient does not match well with common clinical problems, the treating doctors will face a difficulty in maintaining clinical thinking and they need an emergency way of thinking as in this example. By this I mean, any treating doctor needs to change his or her way of thinking to adapt new challenges.

T2 was successful to a certain extent in recognising that this presentation does not match any neurological diseases pattern and for that reason this patient might have a psychological problem or something T2 cannot solve so needs a second opinion.

After reviewing the patient's current and old presentations and knowing his previous medical investigations (including normal brain and Spine MRI), I explained to T2 that this patient will not benefit from the care of a psychologist alone but he needs a pain management program which includes a pain specialist, physiotherapist and psychologist team.

This is an example of having a complaint with no clue as to the reason and therefore needing a second opinion or group of other health practitioners to help, especially when the patient does not trust doctors and accuses them of not being able to solve his problem.

In this scenario, I think I was successful in helping T2 to make thinking broader and try to ask for the help of others' as part of complete management.

The second trainee was quite successful in their use of a non analytic model (pattern recognition) when T2 concluded that the patient's complaint does not fit a neurological deficit and was therefore more likely to be a chronic pain or psychosomatic disorder.

This process of thinking happens when clinicians face patients. They use all possible clues (from history taking or physical examinations or available records) and arrange them in a pattern to reach the diagnosis (Norman et al. 2007). This method is largely dependent on previous knowledge and skills. It is quicker than the hypothetic deductive method since the clinicians will not proceed with all steps of that clinical approach.

T2 attended to the *where* aspect of the problem, and finding no specific evidence for a physical problem, T2 was able to move onto the *what is* the problem.

Story no. 3, "My leg is hurting"

A 56-year-old woman presented with a sore right knee many years ago. She is diabetic, hypertensive and asthmatic. She is on many medications.

Trainee no.3 (T3) was asked to see this patient with me. I attended the consultation as an observer only. We booked a long consultation for this patient as she has many medical conditions.
T3 started taking a history as usual but T3 did not follow a systematic method. Rather, jumping from one subject to another possibly because the patient did not give information easily and changed subjects every now and then. T3 was almost convinced this is a case of osteoarthritis of the knee joint. T3 did not ask about previous history of trauma or any fever that might be relevant to the patient's presentation or pattern of pain.
T3 tried to use a non analytic method (pattern recognition) of clinical reasoning

to reach a diagnosis, however, that did not work. With no clear provisional diagnosis, T3 decided to see this patient later after doing some investigations.

In the second consultation, T3 decided to go back to a standard model of clinical reasoning and utilized an analytic method. T3 found it better and almost came up with more clinical findings and was able to cover most of the diagnostic aspects.

My Observation

This is an example of using a non analytic model of clinical reasoning but when it is aimless, an analytic model proved much more helpful.

In this approach, the young clinicians used both methods (non analytic and analytic) to reach a clinical diagnosis and treatment. They used pattern recognition (non analytic way of thinking) (system 1), when appropriate to reach a diagnosis and, if they can match the pattern, to finalise their management. Otherwise, the analytic method (system 2) (Eva 2002) was the second option to be applied.

Another observation is that it is interesting when you observe others' performance while they are taking history and doing a physical examination. The educator needs to have a few characteristics to be an effective teacher in this situation. I noticed that I needed to be attentive, patient, silent and not interfering at any stage unless the situation called for urgent intervention.

3.3 Trainees' Clinical Approaches

Most of our trainee doctors have a similar clinical approach which is Hypothetical – deductive clinical reasoning (analytic), although sometimes they might change into another approach when they cannot work out what the problem might be. I think they are using this clinical approach because it is the most used method, especially for junior doctors. However, when they build up experience they might change to another method (Eva 2002).

The other observation is, it is not easy for any treating health practitioner to use one single clinical approach in the general practice environment as there are many external factors such as time constraint, an individual patients' presentation, previous knowledge of patients' medical history and other factors.

I noticed as well, some of trainees developed their own approach, for instance, one of the trainees took the time to read previous medical records before seeing the patient and tried to anticipate what the patient would come for. On the other hand, I noticed this approach might be detrimental because those trainees who are preoccupied by some ideas, might be embarrassed when their patients come with different problems which might leave those doctors a bit confused and they go back to first square of Hypothetical – deductive clinical reasoning (analytic).

What I learned from my students!?

Clinical teachers can learn many lessons from their teaching which was very exciting in this journey when I can tell I learned:

> Most junior doctors use Hypothetical – deductive clinical reasoning approach (analytic) when they consult their patients. There are a few possible reasons for this:
> - This method might be a simple and safe one.

- It is the most learned one in medical schools.

I found some of junior doctors try to use a non analytic mode of clinical reasoning and they might succeed in the end but may have some struggles because of a lack of experience with a broad range of examples and then they go back to the analytic method of clinical reasoning.

3.4 Think Anatomy Think Red Flags - Heuristic Approach

This part of thesis comes after recording my first part of findings or observations when I noticed trainees approaching different patients. After the initial experiences, I presented them with the model I use "Think Anatomy, Think Red Flags" and observed them afterwards.

I have spent considerable time assisting patients with chronic pain and spinal disorders. It is not easy to explore the causes of patients' pain since pain is invisible. To identify pain, you need to imagine how it originates and what the reason/s might be, in addition to that the patients' description of pain is crucial. Hence, patients' words might make it more difficult if patients do not have the ability to describe pain well or perhaps a patient might even try to deceive doctors for many reasons including seeking attention or seeking compensation.

It is a skill to correctly identify the reason for any pains and treat that effectively. Moreover, pain might be chronic making it a huge concern for the patient and beyond the capacity of general practice to mange. Therefore, the second opinion of a pain specialist is needed.

In my journey with teaching some general practitioners, I focused on a clinical model to approach a patient with leg pain. However, the approach can be used in upper limbs pain with few modifications.

This model is, generally speaking, a **modification, and bringing together, of many approaches** used by health practitioners to approach a patient with any complaint.

In this thesis, my focus is on approaching a patient with leg pain (acute or chronic) and I used this model to teach students how to classify diseases causing leg pain so I advised them to use anatomical background and relate pain to anatomical structures and then consider which one is the reason of pain or disease. Students should also keep in mind some rare or serious diseases that should not be missed out (I call them Red Flags). **Hence I came up with this heuristic:**

Think Anatomy Think Red Flags

Think Anatomy: means think about where the origin of pain comes from. Consider one or more of the following anatomical structures and then explore what the pathology might be. These structures are: Skin and subcutaneous tissues; Muscles; Joints with ligaments, capsule and tendons; Nerves; Blood vessels (artery or vein); Bone.

Think Red Flags: means to remember some rare or serious or unusual presentations such as: Cancers; Plexitis; Meralgia parasthetica; Paraneoplastic syndrome; Thyroid disorder; Medications or Recreational Drugs side effects; Psychological disease.

Note there might be more Red Flags that can be added by a student when s/he thinks it is necessary. My aim was to enhance the trainee doctor's thinking to be broader and more systematic and not necessarily to be limited to my list.

Other approaches to classifying disease causing leg pain might depend on pathological classification rather than anatomical, as mentioned previously, for instance, when a medical practitioner faces a patient with leg pain s/he will think (is it neoplastic or inflammatory or infectious or psychological or something else). This approach is a valid one but I used my model of thinking to simplify the task and instead of trying remembering the list of diseases I am just asking the trainees to remember the gross anatomy then apply different diseases to it.

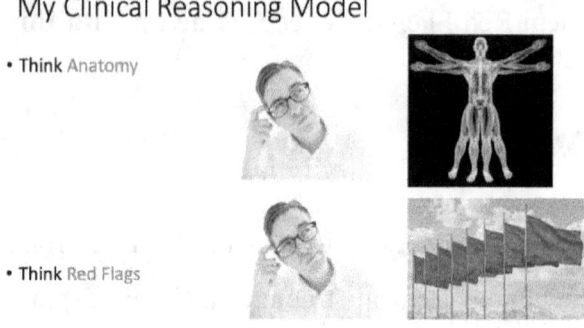

Figure (2) Think Anatomy Think Red Flags

3.5 My Model and Others Models

In the literature review, I outlined some of the main clinical reasoning models used by health practitioners while approaching any clinical problems. My model is similar to the above models in the following ways: It involves the taking of a clinical history from the patient and performing clinical examinations while also collecting all available patients' medical records and examining them.

However, there were a few differences. For example, some models such as the analytic one, mandate thorough history taking and doing clinical examinations to cover all systems then to conclude what the problem might be. In my approach, you need to listen to the patient and while doing so you begin to categorise the problem into anatomical structures and see if it is consistent with one or more of those structures or not. The hypothesis can be further clarified by performing a clinical examination. Secondly, "Red Flags" need to be eliminated.

The approach is less time consuming than others such as the analytic one, it is a modification from the pattern recognition model since there is a focus on recognising the main features of a clinical presentation and excluding others. However, my model is still considering an anatomical way of thinking more than only pattern recognition.

The 'Think Anatomy, Think Red Flags' model is designed for approaching the patient with pain however it might be applied to other complaints if appropriate, and here I will leave it to any health practitioner to decide if it is appropriate or not.

3.6 Few examples after teaching "Think Anatomy Think Red Flags" model:

Note that when I refer to Trainees here, they are not necessarily the same ones as those trainees in first part of the study "before introducing new model". I am discussing only few examples of observations out of the vast amount of data I collected. I am discussing the ones I found the most interesting observations such as finding change of trainee's way of thinking or finding a trainee more efficient in finding a possible diagnosis or some other valuable findings.

Example 1: 43-year-old male patient presented with low back pain radiating to right leg till the big toe with tingling sensation.

Trainee (T4) was able to identify this pattern of pain which is consistent with nerve origin (sciatica), since no other structures can explain this radicular pain except nerves. T4 did not focus on Red Flags but when I asked him about that, he mentioned some and did not pay attention to others because he thought it was an obvious and common presentation, so there was no need to follow all red flags and try to exclude each one.

Overall, I was happy with T4's performance since he was very able to identify pain pattern and used a reasonable clinical reasoning approach although T4 did not mention red flags because, T4 thought the presentations were quite obvious but I think still it is better to follow the principles of Red Flags for a safer approach. However, I appreciate the time pressure factor in the general practice work environment.

Example 2: 72-year-old lady with aching pains in upper and lower limbs.

Trainee (2) (note this trainee is the same one in part one of study) undertook a full detailed history and did a proper clinical examination. I noticed T2 did not have any idea of presentation at the start but later with more detailed history and collecting some information from previous patient's records, T2 was able to assume this pain was coming from muscle origin. This trainee related the patient's complaint and medications history because this patient was using a high dose of statin (which causes myalgia). T2 was able to hypothesise the problem and requested the correct investigation which was a CK (Creatinin

Kinase) blood test to confirm possible diagnosis. When I discussed this case with T2, I noticed that she was almost not paying attention to red flags and even when I asked T2 about any other possibilities but T2 failed to exclude myositis and related cancer pathology.

Example 3: 66-year-old male patient with history of pain moving from back to front of left thigh and groin area. Trainee (5) was able to identify this as a nerve pattern pain but unable to localise which nerve was causing it. This is difficult to diagnose for a junior doctor. The patient has cluneal nerve entrapment (which is not common and not easy to diagnose). The most important observation is that T5 was successful in using a good method of clinical reasoning. At the same time, T5 presented the case to me and was excluding nearly all Red Flags which was impressive.

I am here, very confident that T5 achieved new clinical skills by clarifying pain pattern and excluding other Red Flags but was unable to identify the origin of the pain which is very understandable since it was the first time that T5 had encountered such a medical challenge.

Example 4: 56-year-old lady patient presented with hot feet "I have fire in my feet especially at night".

Trainee (6) was able to assume it is a nerve origin type of pain that is peripheral neuropathy. However, T6 did not proceed further in finding the reason for it when I asked about that.

After further discussion, I reminded the trainee that the patient is not diabetic "because diabetes is one of the most common causes of peripheral neuropathy" and T6 was not sure why I mentioned that.

I then reminded T6 about "Red Flags" and T6 was able to find out that this patient was under chemotherapy and the presentation was most likely a side effects of chemotherapy which causes peripheral nerve damage.

Again the good thing is identifying pain origin by "Think Anatomy" and then the origin of this lesion as "medications" which is part of "Red Flags".

Few observations

After teaching the students my model, I learned new lessons:

- One of the trainees tried to remember this model while *approaching a patient with upper limb pain as well*. He ended up with an idea that it is easy to remember and gave him a better orientation about how to approach such patients.
- I noticed most of students became *more organised* in their history taking and performing clinical examinations. Most of them succeeded in asking enough questions to exclude Red Flags and they undertook better focused clinical examinations for the same purpose.
- One of trainees told me that *this model is almost similar to others* and added not much to him. However, he loved thinking in a more structured way using an anatomical pattern.
- I gave a scenario similar to one of those mentioned above ("my leg is hot") to one of the other trainees. I noticed that *this trainee immediately tried to exclude vascular lesion* in this patient which indicates s/he used this approach at least to be safe.
- It is *interesting* to observe other medical practitioners while they approach a clinical challenge such as pain and try to explore reasons and identify the right management. This *observation stimulated my active thinking further.*
- *Trying to make thinking visible is a very challenging task*, I found it really hard to do that but it is pleasurable when you see your students

happy to explore the diagnosis and can see they are making progress in clinical skills.

One of trainees used a ***diagram for Think Anatomy Think Red Flags*** in the consulting room to assist them to remember. I think this trainee is ***actively thinking and well engaged.***

Another interesting finding is that some of trainees started to ***generalise this approach*** and use it for other clinical problems. For instance, a patient with chest pain. If the beginning medical practitioner applies the same principles (Think Anatomy Think Red Flag) s/he will develop a reasonable and safe clinical approach.

Here, I had a good lesson, why do I not generalise the approach in my own practice? I have noticed that I am doing that sometimes. However, I found it not easy to do in certain situations such as headache since headache should be mostly self-explanatory. When a patient describes their headache clearly, a doctor will usually be able to identify the reason with the aid of lab or imaging studies. However, I am still unsure if this can be applied effectively yet.

Despite that, I think this model can be applied to any place when you think it is possible to remain focused on a gross anatomy and remember rare or serious illnesses. I think most of my trainees used the "Think Anatomy" model very well and this gave them a quick approach for patients with leg pain but they were not very efficient in the second part of the model which is "Think Red Flags". I think this is because of general practice environment factors such as time constraint and lack of experience because they are still under training as junior doctors.

4.0 DISCUSSION

In this chapter, I will discuss different clinical reasoning methods then will discuss my observations before moving to conclusions and recommendations.

This chapter will be divided into two main parts:

I. Different clinical reasoning methods implications.
II. My observations and my model of clinical reasoning in comparison to others.

4.1 Clinical Reasoning Methods Discussion

1. Hypothetical – deductive clinical reasoning (analytic)

In this method of reasoning there are few critical issues to be discussed:

Firstly, there is no clear differentiation between novices' and experts' performance since all of them will follow the same phases in diagnosis, so this method failed to address the capacity of well trained and expert clinician when they approach patients (Yazdani, Hosseinzadeh et al. 2017). However, in my study, the level of trainees is almost similar as being junior level of experience.

Secondly, it is fundamental any clinician have enough knowledge to create diagnostic hypotheses. In other words, the previous fund of knowledge of the clinicians affects the generations of diagnostic hypotheses since they might be more confident and quicker in response to medical problem solving than less knowledgeable clinicians. This approach of clinical reasoning cannot add more clarification to this content related issue of the clinicians, this was stated by Elstein el al as content specificity (Krathwohl 2002, Elstein 2009). I found this to be the case when trainees in this study built knowledge and experience.

Thirdly, this process is usually time consuming which does not fit all types of clinical reasoning since the clinicians might be urged to make a decision quickly despite the lack of enough data from patients. This is particularly the case in emergency situations or in general practice.

The conclusion: this method of clinical reasoning looks like a standard method of cognitive thinking to almost all clinicians but it cannot be the best method for general practitioners who usually face relatively large numbers of patients in a short time frame in comparison to other specialists. Nevertheless, this hypothetic deductive method might be more suitable to junior doctors since it gives them more time and opportunity to think in more detail (Yazdani et al. 2017).

2. Pattern Recognition Method (Non Analytic) of clinical reasoning

There are a few arguments about this type of clinical reasoning:

Firstly, some authors such as Barrows and Feltovich (1987) stated that this non analytic method is in reality a type of analytic (hypothetic-deductive) method of clinical reasoning but is quicker so that the clinicians do not even recognise the process they are using. On the other side, they questioned that the clinicians who are using this pattern recognition method, actually use it only in simple repeated medical problems while they cannot use it in more complicated medical presentations (Findyartini 2012). In most of cases in my study, the trainees were unable to use this method alone because the presentations of pain were usually complicated and in some cases the trainees had no history of encountering the problems.

Secondly, since this method is largely context dependent, this will not be suitable for non experienced trainees or clinicians which will limit the use of this method. This was evident in may of my observations in my study.

Thirdly, this method relies on quick recognition of the patterns without paying much attention to the details and because in medicine there are many differences in clinical problems, the use of this method might result in the trainees missing a few aspects in the management which might increase the chance of mistakes.

The conclusion: this method is useful for many clinicians and especially the general practitioners (Groves et al. 2003) as they might use it to avoid prolonged or unnecessary consultations and be able to move quickly to the next patient. However, mixing this method with the analytic (hypothetic – deductive) method is more suitable in more challenging medical problems to avoid mistakes.

3. **Dual Clinical Reasoning**

There are two critical aspects about this method:

Firstly, this method is mostly used by general practitioners (Balla et al. 2009). Indeed, it is considered one of the favourite methods of general practitioners' clinical reasoning (Yazdani et al. 2017). Nevertheless, in my study, trainees were using the analytic method the most rather this dual model, so this looks different from what is seen by Balla et al (2009) and Yazdani et al (2017). This might be because my study focused on junior levels of general practitioners.

Secondly, this method of dual process is the one mainly employed by cognitive psychologists for that reason there is a lack of enough evidence that this method is the best one to be used by physicians (Sloman 1996).

4. **Pathway for Clinical Reasoning**

The critiques of this method suggest it seems to be non specific and cannot be used easily by beginners or those who are not familiar with it (Yazdani et al. 2017). In addition to that, it is a modification of the hypothetic – deductive method rather than a new method of clinical reasoning (Arocha et al. 1993, Higgs 2008, Atkinson et al. 2011).

5. **Clinical (Diagnostic) Reasoning Strategies Method**

This model depends on stages and strategies to reach the clinical diagnosis, and it did not depend on whether the clinician used an analytic or non analytic clinical approach while facing a clinical challenge. However, this model did not explain how all these stages and strategies work together or should use one of them rather than the other (Yazdani et al. 2017).

6. An Integrative method of clinical reasoning

In this model, the health practitioners depend on two main sources which are (1) their previous knowledge and (2) patients' clinical presentations to formulate an initial representation of the problem before undertaking further evaluations if they fail to reach a diagnosis (Norman et al. 2002). In my study, this model was not used by trainees most likely because they do not have a high experience level.

Additionally, there is no clear way of collecting data from patients whether it is analytic or non analytic. Moreover, the developments of new cycles and evaluation were not clear and might need further clarifications.

4.2 My observations and my model of clinical reasoning in comparison to others.

It was an interesting journey with junior general practitioners while supervising them when they approach their patients. Those general practitioners might consult their patients and then discuss them with me or I might be available at times during consultations. Every time I record my observations and then analyse them.

When I approach a patient with upper or lower limbs pain, I use my prior knowledge in anatomy to organise my thinking so I can imagine what might be the cause of the pain or from where the pain is generated. This needs prior understanding of the anatomy of upper or lower limbs but you do not need to know details, it is simpler than that. This method needs only remembering the major structures namely bone, muscle, joint and its related structures, nerve, vessels, subcutaneous tissue and skin. At the same time, a clinician should not forget the most serious or rare medical problems about which a clinician needs to be vigilant since if these are missed a clinical diagnosis might be late or difficult and will be detrimental to patients.

In comparing my observation to the literature I have found the following:

- The analytic method of clinical reasoning was the predominantly used method by junior general practitioners while others such as Yazdani et al (2017) found the dual method the most widely used. This might be due to the fact that my thesis is about junior doctors rather than more senior ones and in other articles junior doctors are not mentioned (Elstein 2009, Atkinson et al. 2011; Yazdani et al. 2017). However, Elstein found this method is the most commonly used methods by doctors (Elstein 2009)
- Most of our trainee doctors have a similar clinical approach which is Hypothetical – deductive clinical reasoning (analytic), although sometimes they might change into another approach when they cannot find out what the problem is. This might be because they have not built up enough experience to change into another method, this concurs with Eva's findings (Eva 2002).
- Some trainees at certain occasions tried to use an integrative method since they spent a considerable time reviewing a patient's existing data before the consultation. It was not very easy and most of the time they went back to analytic methods of clinical

reasoning. Again this finding is one of argument about integrative methods which were discussed as well by Yazdani et al (2017).

- 'Think Anatomy, Think Red Flags" is a new model used by me to approach a patient with leg pain. However, I use it to approach patients with upper limb and spinal pain too. In this study I focused on leg pain.
- 'Think Anatomy, Think Red Flags" provided most of the trainees with a quick comprehensive method of clinical thinking while approaching patients with leg pain but this thesis did not compare two groups of junior doctors (for instance, one group is using this method and another uses another method). This study might be a call for further studies to compare this model with others in a separate study.
- 'Think Anatomy, Think Red Flags" may not be a good option if a junior doctor faces another medical challenge such as shortness of breath or abdominal pain or even headache since anatomical structures will be different.
- To my best knowledge, I did not find a literature discussing specific clinical reasoning model or method to be used for specific clinical problem, so this method 'Think Anatomy, Think Red Flags" might be a *starting point of using a specific method to a specific clinical challenge.*

5.0 CONCLUSION

There are many methods of clinical reasoning which can be used by general practitioners, each one might suit certain levels of general practitioners' trainees or experts. The use of any of the clinical reasoning methods is affected by the level of the clinicians' experience, the available data, the cultural and social influences in specific situations. There is no one method that is superior in comparison to others, however some methods such as pattern recognition or dual methods are considered more suitable to most clinicians especially general practitioners. In medical challenges such as pain, general practitioners might choose a model like "Think Anatomy, Think Red Flags" since I think this model can be suitable for this specific problem hence it provides a good method of thinking to approach a patient.

Recommendations

- This thesis might be a call for further study to *individualise* clinical reasoning methods to different medical presentations or disciplines in medicine, for instance, clinical reasoning used in approaching a patient with pain differs from that approaching a patient with shortness of breath. For that reason, different specialties such as cardiology, neurology, orthopaedics, pain management and others might have their own clinical reasoning method which can address their need.
- This new model of "Think Anatomy, Think Red Flags" can be used to approach a patient with lower limb pain and might be suitable for spinal pain or upper limb pain. However, this needs further studies.

6.0 REFERENCES

1. Adams, T. E., S. L. Holman Jones and C. Ellis (2015). Autoethnography, Oxford : Oxford University Press, [2015].
2. Adamson, K. A. and S. Kardong-Edgren (2012). "A METHOD and Resoueces for ASSESSING the Reliability of Simulation Evaluation Instruments." Nursing Education Perspectives (National League for Nursing) **33**(5): 334-339.
3. Arocha, J. F., V. L. Patel and Y. C. Patel (1993). "Hypothesis generation and the coordination of theory and evidence in novice diagnostic reasoning." Medical Decision Making: An International Journal Of The Society For Medical Decision Making **13**(3): 198-211.
4. Atkinson, K., R. Ajjawi and N. Cooling (2011). "Promoting clinical reasoning in general practice trainees: role of the clinical teacher." Clinical Teacher(3): 176.
5. Atkinson, P. (1997). Narrative Turn or Blind Alley? Great Britain, SAGE PUBLICATIONS INC: 325.
6. Balla, J. I., C. Heneghan, P. Glasziou, M. Thompson and M. E. Balla (2009). "A model for reflection for good clinical practice." Journal Of Evaluation In Clinical Practice **15**(6): 964-969.
7. Barrows, H. S. and P. J. Feltovich (1987). "The clinical reasoning process." Medical Education **21**(2): 86-91.
8. Borders, L. D. and A. L. Giordano (2016). "Confronting Confrontation in Clinical Supervision: An Analytical Autoethnography." Journal of Counseling & Development **94**(4): 454-463.

9. Ellis, Carolyn, E. A. Tony and P. B. Arthur (2010). "Autoethnography: An Overview." <u>Forum: Qualitative Social Research, Vol 12, Iss 1 (2010)</u>(1).

10. Chang, H. (2016). <u>Autoethnography as Method</u>, Walnut Creek : Taylor and Francis, 2016.

11. Chew-Graham, C. and C. May (1999). Chronic low back pain in general practice: the challenge of the consultation. **16:** 46-49.

12. Collins, J. P. and R. M. Harden (1998). "AMEE Medical Education Guide No. 13: real patients, simulated patients and simulators in clinical examinations." <u>Medical Teacher</u> **20**(6): 508-521.

13. Croskerry, P. (2009). "Clinical cognition and diagnostic error: applications of a dual process model of reasoning." <u>Advances In Health Sciences Education: Theory And Practice</u> **14 Suppl 1**: 27-35.

14. Delany, C. and C. Golding (2014). "Teaching clinical reasoning by making thinking visible: an action research project with allied health clinical educators." <u>BMC Medical Education</u> **14**: 20-20.

15. Delany, C. and E. Molloy (2009). <u>Clinical education in the health professions</u>, Sydney, N.S.W : Churchill Livingston Elsevier, c2009.

16. Downs, M. G., S. Iliffe, S. Turner, J. Wilcock, M. J. Bryans, J. Keady, R. O'Carroll and E. Levin (2004). General practitioners' knowledge, confidence and attitudes in the diagnosis and management of dementia.

17. Macrum E.C (2018). "Problem Based Learning Model Used to Improve General Medical Decision Making." <u>Athletic Training Education Journal (Allen Press Publishing Services Inc.)</u> **13**(1): 82-82.

18. Efron, S. E. (2013). Action research in education : a practical guide, New York Guilford Press, [2013].

19. Egeli, C. (2017). "Autoethnography: A methodological chat with self." <u>Counselling Psychology Review</u> **32**(1): 5-15.

20. Ellis, Carolyn., T. E. Adams and A. P. Bochner (2011). Autoethnography:

an overview, Deutschland, Germany.

21. Elstein, A. S. (2009). "Thinking about diagnostic thinking: a 30-year perspective." <u>Advances In Health Sciences Education: Theory And Practice</u> **14 Suppl 1**: 7-18.

22. Elstein, A. S., L. S. Shulman and S. A. Sprafka (1981). "Medical problem-solving." <u>Journal Of Medical Education</u> **56**(1): 75-76.

23. Emanovský, P. (2015). "PROBLEM-BASED LEARNING AND ITS EFFECT ON LEARNERS' RELATIONSHIPS." <u>Problems of Education in the 21st Century</u> **63**: 53.

24. Eva, K. W. (2002). The Aging Physician: Changes in Cognitive Processing and Their Impact on Medical Practice, Association of American Medical Colleges.

25. Findyartini, A. (2012). Understanding of clinical reasoning and how it is taught and learned in undergraduate medical programs (Australia & Indonesia), 2012.

26. Gardner, K. and D. Mazza (2012). "Quality in general practice: Definitions and frameworks." <u>Australian Family Physician</u>(3): 151.

27. Groves, M., P. O'Rourke and H. Alexander (2003). "The clinical reasoning characteristics of diagnostic experts." <u>Medical Teacher</u> **25**(3): 308-313.

28. Higgs, J. (2008). <u>Clinical reasoning in the health professions</u>, Amsterdam : Butterworth Heinemann, 2008. 3rd ed.

29. Hogan, R. (2013). Autoethnography, Salem Press.

30. Ilgen, J. S., A. J. Humbert, G. Kuhn, M. L. Hansen, G. R. Norman, K. W. Eva, B. Charlin and J. Sherbino (2012). "Assessing diagnostic reasoning: a consensus statement summarizing theory, practice, and future needs." <u>Academic Emergency Medicine: Official Journal Of The Society For Academic Emergency Medicine</u> **19**(12): 1454-1461.

31. Issenberg, S. B., H. S. Chung and L. A. Devine (2011). "Patient Safety

Training Simulations Based on Competency Criteria of the Accreditation Council for Graduate Medical Education." <u>Mount Sinai Journal of Medicine</u> **78**(6): 842-853.

32. Khalil, H. and K. Schliephake (2017). "Design of an online medication safety module for clinicians." <u>International Journal of Evidence-Based Healthcare</u> **15**(2): 63.

33. Kostopoulou, O., B. C. Delaney and C. W. Munro (2008). "Diagnostic difficulty and error in primary care--a systematic review." <u>Family Practice</u> **25**(6): 400-413.

34. Krathwohl, D. R. (2002). "A revision of Bloom's Taxonomy: an overview." <u>Theory into Practice</u>(4): 212.

35. Levine, D. and A. Bleakley (2013). "Rethinking clinical reasoning...Loftus S. Rethinking clinical reasoning: time for a dialogical turn. Med Educ 2012;46:1174–8." <u>Medical Education</u> **47**(7): 745-746.

36. Linn, A., C. Khaw, H. Kildea and A. Tonkin (2012). "Clinical reasoning: A guide to improving teaching and practice." <u>Australian Family Physician</u>(1/2): 18.

37. McAteer, M. (2013). Action research in education, London : Sage, 2013.

38. McBee, E., T. Ratcliffe, K. Picho, A. R. Artino, Jr., L. Schuwirth, W. Kelly, J. Masel, C. van der Vleuten and S. J. Durning (2015). "Consequences of Contextual Factors on Clinical Reasoning in Resident Physicians." <u>Advances in Health Sciences Education</u> **20**(5): 1225-1236.

39. McNiff, J. (2017). Action research : All you need to know, Los Angeles : SAGE, 2017.

40. Méndez, M. (2013). "Autoethnography as a research method: Advantages, limitations and criticisms / La autoetnografía como un método de investigación: ventajas, limitaciones y críticas." <u>Colombian Applied Linguistics Journal</u>(2): 279.

41. Molloy, E. K. and D. Boud (2014). "Feedback Models for Learning, Teaching and Performance." Handbook of Research on Educational Communications & Technology: 413.

42. Monteiro, S. M. and G. Norman (2013). "Diagnostic reasoning: where we've been, where we're going." Teaching And Learning In Medicine **25 Suppl 1**: S26-S32.

43. Morgan, S., G. Ingham, S. Wearne, T. Saltis, R. Canalese and L. McArthur (2015). "Towards an educational continuing professional development (EdCPD) curriculum for Australian general practice supervisors." Australian Family Physician **44**(11): 854-858.

44. Murtagh, J. and J. Rosenblatt (2015). John Murtagh's general practice. [electronic resource], North Ryde, NSW : McGraw-Hill Education, c2015. 6th edition.

45. Norman, G. (2005). "Research in clinical reasoning: past history and current trends." Medical Education **39**(4): 418-427.

46. Norman, G., S. Monteiro and J. Sherbino (2014). "Reflecting upon reflection in diagnostic reasoning." Academic Medicine: Journal Of The Association Of American Medical Colleges **89**(9): 1195-1195.

47. Norman, G., M. Young and L. Brooks (2007). "Non-analytical models of clinical reasoning: the role of experience." Medical Education **41**(12): 1140-1145.

48. Norman, G. R., C. v. d. Vleuten and D. Newble (2002). International handbook of research in medical education / editors, Geoff R. Norman, Cees P.M. van der Vleuten, David I. Newble ; section editors, Geoff R. Norman ... [et al.], Dordrecht ; Boston, Mass. : Kluwer Academic, c2002.

49. Racine, C. A. (2016). Beyond clinical reduction : Levinas, the ethics of wonder and the practice of autoethnography in community mental health care.

50. Ribeiro Bonilauri Ferreira, A. P., R. F. Ferreira, D. Rajgor, J. Shah, A. Menezes and R. Pietrobon (2010). "Clinical Reasoning in the Real World Is Mediated by Bounded Rationality: Implications for Diagnostic Clinical Practice Guidelines." PLoS ONE **5**(4): 1-8.
51. Sloman, S. A. (1996). "The empirical case for two systems of reasoning." Psychological Bulletin(1): 3.
52. Sparkes, A. C. (2000). "Autoethnography and Narratives of Self: Reflections on Criteria in Action." Sociology of Sport Journal **17**(1): 21-43.
53. Stringer, E. T. (2014). Action research, Thousand Oaks, California SAGE, [2014] Fourth edition.
54. Vallente, R. U. P. (2016). Clinical reasoning, Salem Press.
55. Walford, G. (2004). Finding the limits: autoethnography and being an Oxford University Proctor. Great Britain, SAGE PUBLICATIONS: 403.
56. Yazdani, S., M. Hosseinzadeh and F. Hosseini (2017). "Models of clinical reasoning with a focus on general practice: A critical review." Journal Of Advances In Medical Education & Professionalism **5**(4): 177-184.

www.ingramcontent.com/pod-product-compliance
Lightning Source LLC
Chambersburg PA
CBHW060440220526
45465CB00008B/3208